G. S. Petry

A new receipt book for the treatment of all kinds of cancer

Without cutting, burning or loss of blood

G. S. Petry

A new receipt book for the treatment of all kinds of cancer
Without cutting, burning or loss of blood

ISBN/EAN: 9783742833525

Manufactured in Europe, USA, Canada, Australia, Japa

Cover: Foto ©Lupo / pixelio.de

Manufactured and distributed by brebook publishing software
(www.brebook.com)

G. S. Petry

A new receipt book for the treatment of all kinds of cancer

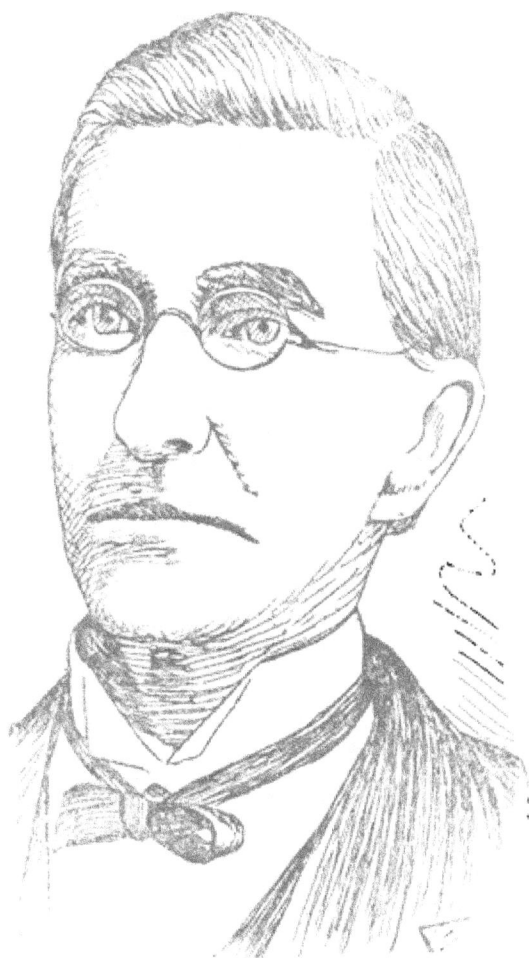

Dr. G. S. PETRY.

A NEW

RECEIPT BOOK

FOR THE

TREATMENT OF ALL KINDS OF

CANCER

WITHOUT CUTTING, BURNING

OR LOSS OF BLOOD.

BY DR. G. S. PETRY,

REDDICK, KANKAKEE COUNTY, ILLINOIS.

STATE OF ILLINOIS, }
  GRUNDY COUNTY, } ss.

I, G. S. **Petry,** do solemnly swear that this book is a complete treatise of my knowledge of curing cancer as practiced by me in my thirty years of experience.

DR. G. S. PETRY

Subscribed and sworn to, before me this **11th** day of April A. D. 1894.   W. S. ALLISON,

Notary Public.

Entered according to act of Congress, in the year 1894,
By DR. G. S. PETRY, REDDICK, ILL.,
In the office of the Librarian of Congress at Washington.

AUTHOR'S PREFACE.

For years past Cancer has been so fatal in its results that the people at large have been led to look upon an affliction of cancer as certain death. The Medical Profession has held nothing more of hope before such suffering victims than the surgeon's knife or a red-hot iron. But cancer originating from a diseased blood does not succumb to a surgical operation as does a wounded or crushed limb. Though driven away for a time it will reappear again when only these external means oppose it. In fact in all my experience of over thirty years I have never found a single instance where a permanent cure of cancer was effected by the use of the knife. Many of the so-called cancers are only common tumors and in such cases an operation is all right and the cure will be permanent. Should any one be skeptical enough on this point to make an investigation he will find the truth of my statement.

For the past 30 years I have successfully treated cancers of all descriptions and stages of development without ever making an operation on the wound or causing the loss of a drop of blood.

Now that I am advanced in years and physically unable to engage in the active practice of medicine, I have concluded to publish, for the benefit of the public, a full and complete account of my system of treatment for all kinds of cancers.

Why die of cancer? It can be cured simply, easily and painlessly as a few of the many testimonials will go to show.

Use Dr. Petry's Cancer Remedy, which effectually and permanently cures all cancers without the surgeon's instruments. If you are suffering from cancer, avoid the tortures of a living death by giving this wonderful remedy a trial. The cure will serve to convince you of its merits. Hoping by the means of this book I may put both remedy and system of treatment in the hands of those so afflicted and thereby be of some service to many of humanity's unfortunates,   I am Cordially Yours,

DR. G. S. PETRY.

Chapter 1.

In my opening chapter I will make a brief survey of the ground I expect to cover and give to the public an adequate idea of this disease in its worst forms and its fatality to the human race.

Cancer like fever appears under different forms and authorities differ on the number of kinds of cancer—some going so far as to put the number at eight others down to five. In my practice of more than thirty years I have come across what I would pronounce seven different varieties. Some noted physicians often call tumors, cancers, which if added would swell the number much larger. These tumors are the *cancers* which the eminent surgeon points to as successfully removed by his knife. True the cure was effected in the proper way but it was no cancer.

Cancer is a disease originating in a bad blood and should receive internal as well as external treatment. It has rightly been styled a dreaded disease, for aside from such terrible diseases as leprosy, etc., no disease is more loathsome than cancer nor produces death more horribly. From some English statistics 1 chanced to read these startling figures of the prevalence of cancer in England alone. In five years the fatalities on that island from cancer was, females 13,783, males 6,426 making a total of over 20,000 deaths by cancer alone in five consecutive years. From this may be seen the extent of this disease. With no adequate treatment these poor unfortunates fall ready victims to the Grim Reaper. I shall consider each kind of cancer, devoting a chapter to symptoms and treatment of each variety.

Chapter II.

Scirrhus or **Hard Cancer** is the first and is perhaps the most frequently met with, being that which we find affecting the breasts of females though by no means confined to this locality alone. After once attacking the breast it is quite likely to be undiscovered until it attains considerable size. Thus before medical advice is sought the disease takes a firm hold upon the system. The Scirrhus cancer is of three varieties—the Acute or Rapid growing; the Chronic or slow growing; the Lardaceous or softer form.

SYMPTOMS.—The general symptoms of Scirrhus cancer consist in the discovery of a hard, unyielding lump which may vary in size from that of a pea to that of a goose egg or larger. At first it is not attended by any pain unless injured in some manner. It generally lies loose in the tissue or part but is sometimes attached to the skin or deeper seated parts of the chest. To the touch it is quite hard and has a rough or nodulated surface, some portions appearing more prominent than others. If closely watched it will be found to steadily increase in size with a greater or less rapidity, if previously loose it will be found to have attached itself although quite loosely. Up to this stage it may be said to be painless and in fact gives rise to irritation of some nerve and this may take place while the tumor is yet small. The pains are not yet constant but are described as of a stinging darting character described by patients as a crawling sensation.

Much indifference on the part of the patient is due from the fact that the pain is not severe and they naturally infer that the disease is not serious, and not until the tumor has attained an inconvenient size do they think of applying for treatment—a most fatal mistake.

The tumor now being of considerable size is composed of a mass of cells, each of which possesses the power of reproduction and multiplication.

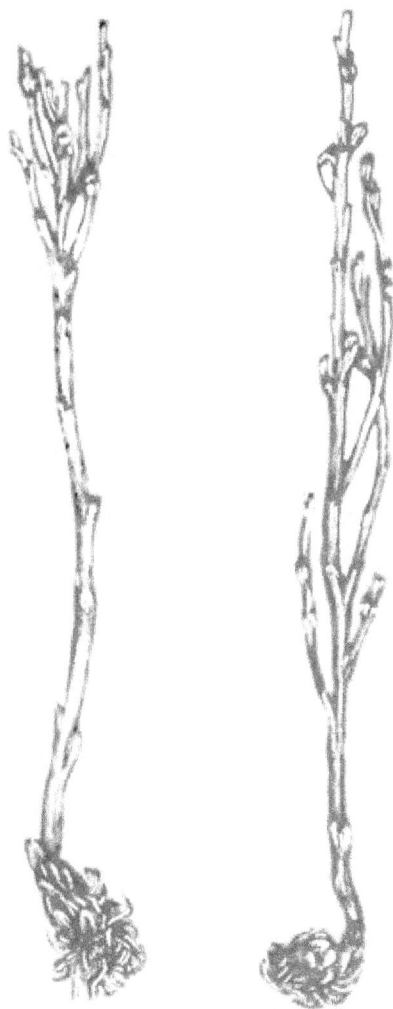

Cancer Root, commonly called "beech drops." (See page 9.)

Internal Treatment.

In all kinds of cancer the internal treatment remains the same throughout.

Cancer powder for internal use.

Flowers of sulphur	2 oz.
Spikenard root	2 oz.
Asafœtida "pulv."	½ oz.
Cream of Tartar	½ oz.

Dose, ¼ teaspoonful, when retiring.

All the above ingredients should be well pulverized and thoroughly mixed into a homogeneous powder.

Cancer Tea, for internal use.

Cancer-root—commonly called beech drops —is found in northern United States and extensively in Canada in large forests and is always found growing at the foot of beech trees, hence the name "beech drops." The plant has a bitter taste and is parasitic, growing on the roots of the beech tree. The plant is leafless, the stem being of a dark or chocolate color. These being gathered root and stem should be dried in the shade and then ground and put in air-tight vessels, keeping it dry and away from the light. The best time of the year to gather the root is in the fall of the year and near full moon, when the plant is most fully charged with sap. This should be done before frost.

In preparation of the cancer tea take three (3) tablespoonfuls of this cancer-root pulverized and one quart of soft water and allow this to simmer [not boil] down to about 1½ pints of the liquid. Then strain off the tea and to the sediment add another pint of soft water and allow to simmer as before down to ½ pint, then strain again. This will give one quart of cancer-root tea which in warm weather must be kept in a cool place, to prevent the liquid from souring. Care should be exercised and only an entirely new vessel be used in which to prepare this tea as it is absolutely necessary that the vessel should be free from oils or grease of every kind.

Directions for internal medicine.

The tea should be taken three times a day, one hour before meals. Dose, one tablespoonful.

The powder should likewise be taken upon retiring. Dose, ¼ teaspoonful as mentioned; the internal treatment as **here** described is used **for all kinds** of cancer to be hereafter spoken of.

External treatment for cancer.

In all cases where the tumor has not yet developed into an ulcer or running sore, apply tincture of Iodine twice a day till the skin cracks open. In case the iodine fails to produce the desired effect the following liniment will be found effectual:—

Oil of Wormwood	½ ounce
Oil of Cedar	2 drams
Oil of Hemlock	2 drams
Oil of Origanum	2 drams
Tinc. Iodine	½ ounce
Alcohol	½ pint.

Mix and apply twice a day as in the case of the iodine. When the surface of the tumor has been cracked open by the application of the iodine or liniment it is then ready to have the cancer salve applied.

Cancer Salve. How made.

Take the sheep sorrel, which has a blue blossom, known also under the name of "Sour Clover," growing generally in new sandy land, gather while plant is in blossom. This should be taken root and stock and extract the juice from it. Place this juice in a clean earthen or porcelain vessel and allow to simmer down un-

til it has the thickness and consistency of apple
butter or thick molasses. It is then ready for
application to cancer. Take a thin white cloth,
rub the surface with cold tallow to prevent the
salve from running through the cloth, then
spread this salve, as thickly as it can be endured,
over the cloth and apply to the cancer. This
salve is to be kept on the cancer during the day-
time only. This salve should be kept away from
the light as when not kept in a dark place it
loses its strength. In case the salve hardens
by age it can be made of the proper consistency
by mixing in a little pure cider vinegar when it
is fresh as new. At night on removing the plaster the cancer should be thoroughly washed in
a strong lukewarm tea, made from the blossoms
of the red clover. After this it should be poulticed for the night. The poultice to be made
from the Red Elm bark ground fine, prepared in
the following manner: Place a sufficient amount,
of the ground Elm bark, to make a poultice
large enough for the cancer, in a vessel and
pour on boiling water. This should then be
stirred thoroughly till it is of the proper thickness for a poultice. Then put the poultice in a
cheese cloth sack and put over the sore. This is

done to prevent the poultice from adhering to the cancer and avoid the difficulty of removing it when dry. The cheese cloth allows the poultice to do its work but at the same time prevents the poultice from sticking to the cancer.

The cancer should thus be poulticed during the night. The cancer salve should be applied by day and the Elm bark poultice by night until the sharp shooting pains have entirely disappeared. Then the healing salve should be applied until the wound is entirely healed over.

Healing Salve. How made.

Take sweet cream and boil it, stirring it continually to keep from burning until the oil and cheese separate. Then take this oil and when cold to about a pint of it add eight or ten drops of Carbolic acid and six grains of White Vitriol. Mix thoroughly and apply this as a salve to the cancer to heal it up. This should be continued until the wound is entirely healed.

Particular notice should here be taken that the external treatment for all cancers is alike with the exception of different salves to be hereafter noticed.

In all cases of cancer three things must be guarded against—Inflammation, Erysipelas and

Exuberant granulation or Proud flesh. When any of these set in the cancer salve ceases to work. This is apt to affect any cancer.

In case of inflammation, if the plant called Live-for-ever can be had, take the leaves, bruise them up and put them on the affected parts. This will serve to reduce the inflammation in a short time. If in the wrong season of the year to obtain it or if otherwise inconvenient make a poultice from buckwheat flour and after it has become cold put it on the inflamed parts. This will be found quite effectual.

If Erysipelas sets in, make an ointment by frying a handful of parsley, root and branch, in a pint of clean lard. Then strain and add a tablespoonful of pulverized camphor gum and it is ready for use. Spread on a cloth and place on the affected parts, leaving it on several hours at a time.

In case of Proud Flesh take burnt alum and brown sugar equal parts and apply. These will be found effectual in all cases.

Chapter III.

Encephaloid, Rose or Soft Cancer. This takes its name from its resemblance, in consistency to the brain. It is the most rapid in growth, attacking various parts of the body and commencing in different forms. When it attacks the breast, like a Scirrhus cancer, it is first noticed as a small lump, which appears to be compressible or elastic causing it to be confounded at times with other kinds of tumors, abscesses or gatherings of the breast. When assuming the acute form its growth is quite rapid, frequently attaining an enormous size in but a few weeks after its first discovery. By their pressure they cause the skin to tighten and become red. The skin soon gives away and a soft fungus growth rapidly protrudes from the orifice resembling Proud flesh. This assumes a great variety of shapes, frequently rolling over on itself in folds thus causing it to be called a Rose cancer. If allowed its own course the tumor culminates in ulceration or sloughing with a profuse and foul discharge. Large masses of the tumor failing longer to receive nourishment slough out leaving an irregular wound often opening blood vessels of sufficient size to cause serious hemorrhage. This form of cancer is especially apt to form about the face as in the eye or on the lips where it first appears as a crack from which this soft elastic growth springs in the form of a button like protuberance. This soon forms into an ulcer, breaks and the cancer begins to affect the surrounding parts.

Treatment.

The internal treatment to be followed is precisely the same as in the case of Scirrhus cancer.

External treatment.

Every morning the cancer should be washed carefully with a strong lukewarm tea made from red clover blossoms. The wound should be evenly dusted with very finely pulverized cancer-root. Then take a pound of California figs and pound them to a pulp. Then place them as a salve upon the cancer. In bad cases where the discharge is profuse the sore must be dressed twice a day with the fig pulp. In most cases every morning is sufficient. At night the sore should be thoroughly cleansed with red clover tea and the Red Elm bark poultice applied precisely as in the case of Scirrhus cancer.

In some cases the fig pulp has been found to be inactive in which case an extract of cranberry juice was found to act very effectively. This is prepared by crushing the cranberries and straining the juice through a cloth to free it of seeds, etc. The juice is then allowed to simmer down in an earthen vessel over a slow fire till it is quite thick. Then allow to cool and it is ready for application. Spread this on a cloth and apply to the cancer as in the case of the fig pulp.

When the pains have entirely disappeared it is an evidence that the cancer is dead and for a healing ointment use the cream salve as in the foregoing case. Continue until the wound is completely healed over.

Chapter IV.

Another variety of cancer is called the Colloid and is not so frequent as the ones just mentioned. Some medical authorities do not acknowledge this as a distinct variety of cancer but class it among Recurrent Tumors.

Colloid cancer is not so often met with on the surface of the body but is more frequently found internally located in the bowels or stomach. Its characteristic feature is that it is composed of cells which are filled with a gelatinous matter like honey in the comb.

Internal treatment.

Use the cancer tea and powder as prescribed in the first case.

External treatment.

Make a wash of one gill of brandy, two tablespoonfuls of salt and 20 drops of carbolic acid and bathe the sore three times a day. After bathing, dust the sore with finely pulverized cancer-root. Then cover the sore with a cloth spread thinly with mutton tallow. After the cancer has been destroyed, heal up the wound with the cream salve.

Chapter V.

Melanosis or Black Cancer is another variety occasionally met with. It closely resembles the Encephaloid cancer in its manner of growth and general character. Its peculiarity and distinguishing characteristic is that it is composed of cells filled with a large quantity of black coloring matter. It will not readily be mistaken for any other variety as it is much darker than any of the rest.

Internal treatment.

Identical with the foregoing.

External treatment.

Take the yolk of a fresh egg and an equal amount of pulverized table salt and a similar quantity of garlic pulverized fine. Mix these thoroughly into a paste to apply to the cancer.

Wash the cancer with the strong lukewarm tea of red clover blossoms and then apply the above paste as a salve. This is to be applied daily and at night put on the Red Elm bark poultice previously described. When the cancer has been killed, heal the wound over with the cream salve as in other cases of cancer.

Chapter VI.

We are now to treat of another cancer known as the Epithelial or Cutaneous. This is the kind that generally attacks the skin or mucus membrane without first giving rise to any tumor. If there is any evidence of its presence it is in a small wart and is attended with little or no pain. It is generally found near some of the natural outlets of the body as the nose, mouth, etc., but is also frequently met with upon the skin of the hand, body or face. It is noticed under a variety of forms in its beginning. It may appear as a small pimple which soon breaks down leaving an ulcer with high edges and rapidly spreading cavity. It may originate as a mere crack in the lip or nose which is only considered as a cold sore until it has made considerable progress. This soon forms into an eating ulcer. Sometimes it is first found as a mere scab which loosens and peels off discharging a sticky matter forming another scab, but each time larger than before until it becomes an open ulcer.

Another form is that of a Scirrhus wart which is first taken to be a seed wart, but soon begins to get sore and maturates when it becomes an ulcer. These all possess the power of affecting the surrounding glands, spreading in them the same disease and we have a fully developed cancer.

TREATMENT. Internal medicine is the same in this case as in all others, the tea and powder.

External treatment.

When the scab has dropped off, apply equal parts of extract of strawberries and extract of cranberries and turpentine, mixed, making a kind of salve. Apply this during the day and at night use the Elm bark poultice. When there is no more tendency to form a scab the cancer is dead and the sore should be healed over by the use of the cream salve. This is the last of the external cancers and now we come to those which affect the internal organs.

Chapter VII.

Cancer of the Stomach or Bowels.

Unlike cancers on the surface of the body the internal cancer is only apparent from its symptoms and cannot be seen like the former.

The first evidences of an internal cancer is that the patient experiences an oppressive sensation in the stomach after meals. Rich foods cause a more distressing feeling than any other. Strong coffee is especially distressing as is vinegar and sour foods. As the cancer progresses the symptoms are similar to those of dyspepsia and is often mistaken by physicians for dyspepsia. The patient spits up particles of food and feels as if a hard lump was in the stomach. This keeps on progressing and intense pain is produced until a few hours before death it ceases and vomiting sets in and the patient dies.

Treatment.

Nothing in the way of drink should be taken into the stomach except Red Clover tea [made from red clover blossoms] cancer tea and sweet milk.

In the way of foods nothing except cracker soup, oyster soup, rice, fresh fish, oatmeal should be eaten. Caution against eating too much should be taken. It is better to take a little at a time and four or five times a day.

Directions.

The cancer tea should be taken in tablespoonful doses three times a day, one hour before meals. Take a teaspoonful of extract of sheep sorrel, add one drachm of Magnesia-calcined and dissolve it in about a pint of cold water and take a tablespoonful of this mixture three times a day, two hours after meals. In case the extract of sheep sorrel produces a bad effect on the stomach as it does with some persons, causing vomiting, this should be replaced by extract of cranberries prepared in the same way and taken under the same directions.

Careful attention should be paid to the internal medicine in all kinds of cancer as my experience has taught me that it is far more important than the external as it reaches the seat of cancer—the blood.

Chapter VIII.

At the close of this short work on cancers it may be well to mention a few of the many causes which produce these terrible sores. Many times in my practice I have been asked what causes these cancers so I will take a short space here to discuss that briefly. In all my experience every case of cancer on a female's breast could be traced to a bruise or to tight lacing, with the exception of a single instance where it was caused by milk drying in the breast making a nucleous from which the cancer began to grow. But the majority of all cancers originate from poisonous blood which is caused in many ways.

The blood may be made impure in many ways as impure air and impure foods taken into the system but I will mention one way especially which poisons the blood, that is the eating of articles and fruits canned up in tin cans which by their natural acids attack the tin thus poisoning the contents and when this is taken into the system it gradually poisons the blood and cancer is the natural result. Too much care can not be exercised in the selection of foods which are free from these poisons. The large proportion

of cancer cases occurring in the city where fruit
canned in tin cans is extensively used is indic-
ative of something. And I believe many of our
cancer cases might be traced directly to this
source. Of course not all foods put up in tin
cans become poisonous but only those which
have an acid that attacks the tin. It can readily
be detected whether foods are in danger of being affected, by examining the inside of the
can. If it is bright the food is all right but if
the surface is tarnished it shows evidence of acid
acting upon it and it is unsafe to use it.

Chapter IX.

In closing I wish to add a few words on
the care to be exercised by patients themselves.
It is exceedingly important that one suffering
from cancer should be very careful of his diet
and habits of life.

In drink especially should the patient guard
himself. He should abstain from the use of
strong drink and all kinds of liquor. Sweet
milk and chocolate is the best drink that can be
used, and may be taken quite extensively. It is
almost an impossibility to effect a cure of cancer on a patient who is addicted to strong drink,

the tobacco habit or the opium or morphine habit. These must be dispensed with if the patient hopes to become cured of his cancer. Only the most wholesome foods should be taken into the system and the patient should guard against overheating the blood or contracting cold. If the utmost care is used by the patient and the treatment as prescribed is carefully followed the cure of almost any cancer is a simple matter.

Chapter X.

In the closing chapter I will add a few of the many testimonials in my possession to show the practical effects of this system of cancer treatment. It will be seen that these are all reliable parties who are ready to testify to the merits of the cancer cure as set forth in this little book.

MARSEILLES, La Salle Co., Ill., April 19th, 1878.

I owe more than my humble thanks to Dr. G. S. Petry for the remarkable cancer cure he effected on my face. It was considered a very bad cancer and pronounced incurable. It affected my whole system and I had been treated by other cancer physicians. I was in a cancer hospital in Chicago for some time and had the cancer cut out, but all to no avail. I had given up all hopes of being cured, when I was persuaded to try Dr. Petry, and he cured me without cut, burn or loss of blood. I would cheerfully recommend Dr Petry to all who suffer from cancer.

JOSEPH FERTIG.

GARDNER, Grundy Co., Ill., March 27, 1879.

DR. G. S. PETRY,

Dear Sir:—I feel more than thankful to you for curing a lump on the under lid of my eye which was pronounced a bad cancer of more than six years standing. Many physicians called it a cancer and advised me to have it cut out immediately to save my eye, and I employed one physician who burned it out with caustic. It healed over but in a few weeks commenced to grow faster than ever. Under Dr Petry's treatment it has been entirely cured for over nine months and no signs of its return to this day.

Respectfully yours,

S. DLAMATTER.

CABERY, Ford Co.. Ill.. April 28, 1878.
Thanks alone would be an insufficient remuneration to Dr. G. S. Petry for his successful treatment of cancer on my face without the use of a knife, searing iron, or causing the loss of a drop of blood. The entire treatment was attended with very little pain. I can recommend Dr. Petry.

MARYANN IMHOFF.

GARDNER, Grundy Co., Ill., June 3, 1880.
This is to certify that my wife was a sufferer of cancer in her nose and she is now completely cured by Dr G. S. Petry. No cutting, no burning, no loss of blood and very little pain. I would advise any one suffering with cancer to try Dr. G. S. Petry's remedy.

J. H. KAUFFMAN.

GARDNER, Grundy Co., Ill., March 24, 1879.
Thanks cannot express my gratitude to Dr. G. S. Petry for his successful cancer cure effected on me. I had a cancer on my nose for twenty-four years and now I am completely cured, and it was accomplished without cutting, burning, or loss of blood.

MATILDA SNYDER.

SAN FRANCISCO, Cal., June 27, 1880.
DR. G. S. PETRY,
Dear Sir:—I have a friend here that has a cancer on his face the same as I had which your medicine cured without cutting or burning. The doctors all call it a cancer. If you will please send me $5.00 worth of the same medicine you sent me I will send you the money. Yours truly,
61, 62, & 63, Col. Market.   S. T. PIKE.

FORD P. O., Ford Co., Kansas, May 30, 1880.
DR. G. S. PETRY,
Sir:—The cancer on my lip is cured by your medicine and I owe my thanks to you for the successful cure of my lip. Yours truly,

I. FORD.

HIGHLAND, Ill , July 19, 1880.

I wish to express my gratitude to **Dr. G. S.** Petry for curing my wife of a cancer on her neck. It was called by some of the best doctors the worst kind of **a** cancer and now it is completely cured. The cure **was** effected without cutting, burning or loss of blood, **and** was attended with no pain, and entirely healed **up in** six weeks. I would recommend all sufferers of **cancer** to **Dr. Petry** whose **success** in treatment of **cancer is** unbounded. U. R. **ELLIS.**

BEAVERDAM, Kosciusko Co., Ind., Nov. 1, 1886.

For the benefit of all those suffering **with cancer,** I write the following:

About nine months ago my mother **had a** very bad cancer on her leg and was treated by **a cancer** doctor, getting **worse** all the time. He then pronounced it an incurable **cancer.** We then **sent** for Dr. G. S. Petry, who called **it** an Insidious cancer and **began** treatment. In four days all the inflammation **and** pain was gone and in six weeks she was entirely **well** and has been well since. Yours,

JOHN KUHN.

JOLIET, Will Co., Ill., Aug. 24, 1878.

DR. G. S. PETRY,

Dear Sir:—I owe more than my thanks **for** curing a cancer on my daughter's face. A physician in **Mt.** Carroll, Ill., pronounced it a Rose cancer and burned it out with acid but did not cure it. I then applied to Dr Petry, who called it a Scirrhus cancer and his remedy cured it **in** a short time.

REV. **L. WILLEMAN.**

CABERY, Illinois, Aug. 4th, 1894.

Eleven years ago Dr. Petry of Reddick, Ill., cured a cancer on the left side of my face. It has never shown any sign of returning and my general health has been good since. Yours for suffering humanity,

MRS. S. J. ELLIOTT.

NEVADA, Illinois, December 15, 1884.

To all whom it may concern:—I hereby certify that a cancer on my nose and a part of my upper lip, of 18 years standing, having destroyed my nose and upper lip, has been completely cured by Dr. G. S. Petry. I had been treated by many other physicians who pronounced it as incurable, and had spent much money in vain. It is now perfectly cured by Dr. Petry without either cutting or burning. I give my gratitude to him, and for his benefit as well as for the good of other sufferers of cancer, I give this certificate in good faith. GEORGE MARTIN.

I am the mother of the above George Martin and hereby certify that the above is true.

MRS. MARY MARTIN.

NAPERVILLE, Ill., April 21, 1894.

I will now make known to the public that I have been troubled with a sore ankle for twenty-five years. It was a veriuse ulcer. Some doctors called it King's Evil. I have spent hundreds of dollars and found no cure until I met Dr. G. S. Petry of Reddick, Ill., and used his medicine. Now I am well and my ankle is cured and for a small sum.

B. F. BENDER.

STREATOR, La Salle Co., Ill., Nov. 22, 1890.

A remarkable success, for ten months ago I was very sick. I had a very bad cancer in my breast. It had gone so far that I gave up all hopes of recovering. I went to two doctors in Streator and both told me that the breast had to be taken off. Both are prominent doctors and one of them said he would take the case in hand for $150. Through the providence of God Dr. G. S. Petry, of Reddick, Ill., came along and cured me without cutting or burning or loss of blood. I can recommend Dr. Petry, of Reddick, with all confidence to any one who may be afflicted as I was.

MRS. S. HOOD BROCKFORD.

South Streator, Ill.

COLUMBUS, Cherokee Co., Kan., **April 25, 1894.**
This is to certify that in 1892 I had a **sore** on the **side** of my face and the doctors in Columbus examined me and all said it was a cancer and they wanted to cut it out, but I would not give my consent to it. Dr. G. S. Petry, of Reddick, Ill., removed it without cutting or burning or loss of blood and without pain. I feel indeed grateful to the doctor for his successful **cure.**

EDWARD BLINCO.

BRADEWOOD, Ill., Oct. 14th, 1893.

I have the pleasure of saying **that I** was healed of a cancer on my face of about nine years standing, by the help of God and through Dr. G. S. Petry, of Reddick, Ill. His cancer remedy healed me in about seven **weeks without** cutting or burning it **out.**

ANNA E. SMITH.

MAZON, Grundy Co., Ill., March 12, 1883.

Dr. G. S. PETRY:—I **owe** you, **my** dear friend, **a** thousand thanks for your success **in** curing a cancer on my wife's hand after employing several doctors who finally concluded that the hand must be taken off. Following the advice of one of my neighbors I employed Dr. Petry and her hand **was** entirely cured in less than six weeks without **cutting,** burning or loss of blood and without any **pain. I ad**vise any one who suffers from cancer to go **to Dr. G. S. Petry.**

Sulphur Springs, Ill.   GEORGE HEROLD.

GARDNER, Illinois, June 1, 1894.

We feel **it** our duty to **make known to** the **public** and suffering community at large that the Rev. **Co**dey, at one time pastor of the Baptist Church here, after being operated on twice with the knife for the **cure** of a cancer of the lip, and proving unsuccessful, **was** duly cured by Dr. Petry without the aid of a **knife or** being burned.

WM. L. SMITH, Pharmacist.
J. H. MELHUISH, Pharmacist.

GARDNER, Ill., Dec. 1, 1888.

This is to certify that I was cured of a cancer on my ankle in the year 1887 by the use of medicine prescribed for me by Dr. G. S. Petry of Reddick, Ill. I am sixty-six years old and have the best of health and can truly recommend Dr. G. S. Petry's remedy to the public.   CHLOE BOOTH.

NAPERVILLE, Ill., April 10, 1894.

DR. PETRY,

Dear Sir:—I am very thankful and pleased for the opportunity of informing you and the public of the cure you effected on me. I would advise all who are suffering from old sores to call on Dr. Petry of Reddick, Illinois. For twelve years I suffered with a sore on one of my ankles. It discharged matter from twelve different places and I went about on crutches all that time and my leg wasted half away and it was hardly ever free from pain. Dr. Petry was in Naperville attending a few cancer cases and I was advised by a friend to let him examine my ankle. I told him it was useless as I had 17 different doctors at work on it up to the present time. My friend insisted and I finally called on Dr. Petry. I found his charges so light that I took treatment from him two months. At the end of that time I left my crutches in the back yard and have had no use for them since. In a short time my ankle was perfectly sound, all of which I owe to Dr. Petry. Yours very respectfully,

G. W. DECKER.

Chapter XI.

I will add at the close of this **little book** some valuable receipts which I have found to be **very** effective in many cases which I have met in my many **years of** practice. They form no part of the treatise **on cancer,** but are **rather a** supplement to **it.** I give them to the public at this time because it is very convenient at the **issuing** of my cancer work to add a few pages **and it may serve to benefit some of my patrons. Among these receipts will be found other meth- ods of treating cancer, the use of which I only advise when my previous** remedies **have been given a thorough trial.** My experience **has taught me that it** is rarely if ever **necessary to resort to any** other treatment than **that pre- scribed in the** fore part of this work.

There are also other cancer remedies recom- mended of which we will name a few:

One is—take yellow **dock root and boil it** in soft water and wash the **sore with it.**

Another **is to put on crushed cranberries,** changing every six hours.

Another, put table salt in the best brandy, **as much** salt as it will dissolve, and wash the **sore with it.**

Another, take a handful of beech drops and four stems of Live-for-ever root (commonly called so), blood root two tablespoonfuls, placed in a clean crock, and pour in two quarts soft water and simmer down in the crock to one pint then add to it about three ounces of fresh butter, and bees wax the size of a walnut and simmer down until the juice is all evaporated, then it is ready for use.

Another, take alum one ounce, borax one ounce, cow urine four gallons, boil down to one gallon and wash the sore four times a day.

Cure for Rose Cancer.

Take good ripe tomatoes, slice them and apply to the sore three times a day, and keep this up till the roots are all dead. Then apply the healing salve.

Good Poultices.

(*a*) Take white beans one pint, cook and mash, and add one teaspoonful saleratus and apply to the sore.

(*b*) Take the roots of garden carrots 2 ounces, flour of Red Elm bark half-ounce, boiling water sufficient to form a poultice. Used on tumors and painful sores.

(c) Take pulverized charcoal and common baker's yeast a sufficient quantity to form a poultice; or take pulverized charcoal one **ounce**, powdered flaxseed 2 ounces, common Elm poultice one pint, **and** soaked bread one teacupful ; **mix and stir well. If it is** too thick **add hot water.**

To Relieve Pain

and inflammation in cancer treatments, take a heaping **teaspoonful of the compound, powder** of Jalap, **which may be mixed with half this** quantity of **cream of tartar and a gill of water. If necessary, repeat in two or three days.**

Whenever fever is in the sore, stop using the salve and apply poultice of slippery elm or starch until the fever is out.

Caution to Patients.

First use very little salt in your food, and no vinegar at all or any spirits, or tobacco. *Beware of using any fruit put up in tin fruit cans as it is blood poisoning.*

For Tumors

I use the following,

Iodine	$\frac{1}{2}$ dr.
Alcohol	1 oz.

mix and apply twice a day with a feather, till

the skin commences to crack, then apply once a day or every other day.

Or	Oil of Wormwood	4 dr.
	Oil of Cedar	2 dr.
	Oil of Hemlock	2 dr.
	Oil of Amber	2 dr.
	Oil of Origanum	2 dr.
	Alcohol	$\frac{1}{2}$ pt.

Wash twice a day.

Salt Rheum.

First use some good blood cleansing medicine and then apply the pure pine tar in the way of a plaster, completely covering the sore, and let it remain nine days. When removing the plaster saturate the cloth with fish oil until it is easily removed. Then wash the sore with sulphur soap and apply cod liver oil as a healing ointment. Cleanse every day by washing with the sulphur soap. The cod liver oil is best applied on oil paper as a cloth absorbs too much of the oil. Keep up this treatment until the sore is healed, giving the limb as much rest as possible.

For Gangrene.

Take one pill of bichlorid, dissolve in one pint water, and wash the sore three times a day—and internally take port wine and peruvian bark, the compound **wine of** comfrey, or carbonate of ammonia, etc., being careful not to administer these stimulants as long as any inflammatory symptoms remain and the pulse **is** strong.

For Melanosis **or** Black **Cancer.**

Take equal parts of arsenic, charcoal made from **black** alder, and ashes from dog **wood.** Wet the cancer on the center, put as much **of** the compound on **the wet place as can be held on the póint of a pen knife.** Place **a thin piece of cloth over the cancer and** wet with the **yolk of an** egg **to** make it **stick.** Press and apply **every** day, always put powder on center of **cancer.** If too painful put poultice of Live-for-ever **or** bread and sweet milk over the other plaster.

A Remedy

for Cancers, Tumors, Carbuncles, Swellings, Sore Throat, Ulcerations of the Mouth, **Indolent** Ulcers, Ophthalmia, Boils and all Painful Tumors, Scrofula of the Womb, Gravel **and** Bleeding of the Kidneys, and Ulcerations **of the** Bladder:—Take the round leaved Pyrola. **This is** a perennial evergreen shrub, common in

various parts of the U. S., bearing numerous
white flowers in June. It is also known by the
names, Pear Leaf, Wintergreen, Canker Let-
tuce, Shin Leaf. The herb is tannic ; it has been
used in decoction both externally and internally.
DOSE :—From one to six grains of the extract
repeated three or four times daily. Externally
the decoction will be found an excellent local
application in sore throat.

Epithelial or Cutaneous Cancer,

by some called Spider Cancer, commences with
a brown spot under the skin, and through a
magnifying glass you can see the roots which
look like spider legs.

(1). For external use take one pint of olive
oil, and put in a bottle with about 25 spiders ;
cork tightly and hang in the sun till they are all
dissolved, then add three tablespoonfuls of gun-
powder and one teacupful of brown sugar and
apply three times a day.

(2). Take turpentine one ounce, and oil of
camphor one ounce, and potassa of bicarbonas
one ounce, and the juice of poke berries one
pint; mix and add flowers of sulphur enough to
make a salve. If you can't get the poke berries
take the juice of cranberries.

A certain cure for the bite of Mad Dogs and other Animals.

DIRECTIONS:—For one person take a quart of Strong Beer, and one ounce of Redchick Weed; put it into a clear earthen vessel and boil it over coals till it is reduced one-half; take one ounce of Venice Treacle, or Teriac as it is sometimes called, put it in, stir it well, and strain it boiling hot through a piece of clean linen into a pewter dish. Let it stand till it is lukewarm. Bottle it, and use as follows: If the person bitten is of a strong constitution, the whole dose must be given at three equal draughts; all doses must be taken according to the constitution of the patient. For a growing person of a weak constitution, a gill every morning, for three mornings, is sufficient. For a child of 12 years of age, one-half the quantity of each kind is sufficient; the whole measure of Beer to be taken. A small child requires less.

A beast must have an ounce of each kind taken at a dose; keep your beast from water or anything greasy for two weeks. Rye-bran and water may answer for drink to be given cold. The medicine must be warmed in a clear vessel.

If persons have already got the malady, and cannot take the medicine without assistance, those giving the medicine, must be cautious of the breath of the diseased—for it is dangerous to catch. The medicine is to be taken in the morning, after fasting several hours; abstain from fresh water; a little wine and water may be taken, but not immediately after taking the medicine. The day on which the medicine is taken, a pancake baked in butter may be taken for dinner. The cloths which the person was bitten in ought to be buried or burned. The wounds must be well washed out at a running stream, with an oak stick with some of the medicine for several days.

For healing the wound, any drawing salve is sufficient. After using the medicine the patient must abstain about two weeks from eating anything that contains pork or baked in lard. Water fowls and fish must not be eaten; all sorts of cabbage, sour and sweet beans or peas must be abstained from for two weeks; gentle sweating is very beneficial. The patient must be cautious against overheating himself or getting angry. By following these directions the medicine will cure even when already mad, after the first and second fit or malady.

A Remedy for Hydrophobia.

The time between the biting of an animal by a mad dog and the showing signs of hydrophobia is not less than nine days but may be nine months. After the animal has become rabid, a bite or scratch with his teeth upon a person, or slabber coming in contact with a sore or raw place, would produce hydrophobia just as soon as though he had been bitten by a mad dog. *Hydrophobia can be prevented*, and I will give you what is known to be an infallible remedy if properly administered, for man and beast; a dose for a horse or cow should be four times as great as for a person. It is not too late to give the medicine any time before the spasms come on. The first dose for a person is 1½ oz. Elecampane root, bruised, put in a pint of new milk, reduced to one half by boiling, then taken all at one dose in the morning, fasting until afternoon, or at least a very light diet after several hours have elapsed. The second dose the same as the first, except take 2 oz. of the root ; third dose same as the last, to be taken every other day. Three doses are all that are needed, and there need be no fear.

This I know from my own experience; and I know of a number of other cases where it has been entirely successful. This is no guess work. Those persons to whom I allude were bitten by their own rabid dogs, that had been bitten by rabid dogs, and were penned up to see if they would go mad ; they did go mad and did bite the persons. This remedy has been used in and about Philadelphia 40 years or longer, with great success, and is known as the Goodman remedy. I am acquainted with a physician who told me that he knows of its use for more than 30 years, and never knew a case that failed where it was properly administered. Among other cases he mentioned, one was where a number of cows had been bitten by a mad dog ; to half the number they administered this remedy, to the other half, not ; the latter all died with hydrophobia, while those that took the Elecampane and milk showed no signs of the disease. R. C. SHOEMAKER.

Montgomery Co., Pa.

VALUABLE RECEIPTS

Proved by DR. G. S. PETRY and Others.

WHOOPING COUGH.

Raw linseed oil one half pint, honey one half pint, brandy or rye whiskey one half pint, boil. Dose, one teaspoonful three times a day.

JAUNDICE.

Jaundice root one ounce pulverized. Dose, one fourth teaspoonful twice a day.

SORE EYES.

Snow or rain water one pint, white vitriol one drachm, rock candy one ounce. Filter through silk paper, wash morning and evening.

RHEUMATISM OR NEURALGIA.

Pure rye whiskey one quart, pure white pine gum one ounce, black cohish one ounce. After dissolved, dose one tablespoonful in water before or after meals.

ERYSIPELAS, ITCH, IVY POISON, OLD SORES.

One pint of clean lard, parsley root and stock one handful, camphor gum pulverized one tablespoonful. Fry and strain then ready to use.

FELONS.

Slack lime in soft soap, spread thick on a rag then wrap over felon ten to fifteen minutes before felon is open.

CHAFING IN CHILDREN.

Subnitrate of bismuth, tie a small quantity in a coarse flannel rag and dust the chafed parts. Or take compound of cabeum tooth powder. Dermal powder.

BURNS.

Equal parts lard, raw linseed oil, mutton tallow, bees wax, melt and mix.

RUN AROUND.

Wrap the finger in cotton batting until healed.

CATARRH.

Citric acid in one pint rain water, syringe twice a day.

MAGIC LINIMENT.

To one pint hot drops made with alcohol, add two ounces each, oil of sassafras, oil of hemlock, spirits of turpentine and camphor, and one ounce each of oil of origanum and oil of cinnamon, when made add lard oil or linseed oil, one sixth part of the whole bulk or about one gill. This forms a valuable liniment in sprains, bruises, rheumatism, neuralgia, or wherever a liniment is needed.

BLOOD PURIFIER.

Iodide of potassium, from two to ten grains in cold water twice a day.

LINIMENTS.

For internal or external use:

Alcohol	1	qt.
Oil of Sassafras	1	oz.
Oil of Origanum	1	oz.
Oil of Peppermint	$\frac{1}{2}$	oz.
Camphor	$\frac{1}{2}$	oz.
Chloroform	2	dr.
Capsicum	2	oz.
Ether of Sulphuric	$1\frac{1}{2}$	oz.

Dose: From 5 to 25 drops in cold water for internal use and for external bathe the parts afflicted. This liniment is good for all kinds of pains.

LIGHTNING OIL.

For internal and external use. Cramp Colic, Diarrhea, Cholera, Rheumatism, Neuralgia, Toothache and sores:

Oil of Sassafras	1½ oz.
Oil of Cinnamon	1 oz.
Oil of Wintergreen	1½ oz.
Camphor	½ oz.
Assafetida	½ oz.
White Glue	½ oz.
Capsicum	8 gr.

Mix and put in a bottle, cork tightly and set in warm place for ten days, shaking it frequently.

PAIN LINIMENT.

Maple Molasses	1 teacup
Yellow Sugar	1 teacup
Strained Honey	1 teacup
Glycerine	1 teacup
Sweet Oil	1 teacup
Carbolic Acid	1 teaspoonful or 30 drops

Mix cold and shake each time before using.

LINIMENT FOR SWELLING FEVER SORES OR RUNNING SORES.

Alcohol	1 pt.
Sweet Oil	1½ oz.
Castor Oil	1½ oz.
Rain Water	½ pt.
Pulverized Borax	2 dr.

Put the alcohol, sweet oil and castor oil together and let stand until well mixed before putting in the water and the borax.

Remedy for sores caused by lye or acids. Wash with pure cider vinegar.

DIARRHEA.

Alcohol	1 qt.
Oil of Origanum	1 oz.
Oil of Sassafras	1½ oz:
Oil of Peppermint	4 dr.
Gum Camphor	3 dr.
Tincture of Capsicum	4 oz.
Sulphuric Ether	12 dr.
Chloroform	2 dr.

Mix. Dose: Half teaspoonful three times a day.

CROUP.

Raw Linseed Oil	1 qt.
Oil of Cedar	2 dr.
Oil of Sassafras	3 dr.
Oil of Hemlock	3 dr.
Oil of Origanum	1½ oz.
Tincture of Lobelia	1 dr.

Mix. Dose: ½ teaspoonful every 2 hours until better. During croup keep hands and feet warm and the neck cold.

RHEUMATISM. For Internal use.

Old Rye Whiskey	1 qt.
Flower of Sulphur	2 oz.
Cream of Tartar	2 oz.
Saltpeter	½ oz.
Snakeroot	¼ oz.
Gum Quack	¼ oz.

Dose: One tablespoonful twice a day.

AGUE.

Alcohol	1 pt.
Quinia	20 gr.
Tincture of Rhubarb	25 gr.
Capsicum	20 gr.
Myrrh	20 gr.

Dose: 1 teaspoonful 3 times a day in cold water.

GOLDEN SEAL.

Raw Linseed Oil	1 qt.
Oil of Cedar	2 dr.
Oil of Origanum	2 dr.
Oil of Sassafras	3 dr.
Oil of Hemlock	2 dr.
Gum of Camphor	$\frac{1}{2}$ oz.

Dose: 1 teaspoonful. It is good for coughs, colds, or pains in the bowels or the stomach.

CHOLERA BALM.

Alcohol	1 pt.
Spirits of Camphor	3 oz.
Tincture of Opium	$\frac{1}{2}$ oz.
Tincture of Capsicum	1 oz.
Syrup of Ginger	$\frac{1}{2}$ oz.
Peppermint	4 oz.

Dose: One teaspoonful.

FOR CANCER AND OTHER SORES.

Rain Water	4 gal.	Borax	2 oz.
Aloes	2 oz.	White Vitriol	2 oz.

Mix and boil down to one gallon. Wash the sore with this twice a day.

ALL KINDS OF SORES.

Soft Water	1 pt.	Castor Oil	1 pt.
Alcohol	1 pt.	Borax	1 oz.
		Balsam of Tolu	4 oz.

To be used externally.

OLD SORES.

Yellow of two raw eggs.	
Pulverized Charcoal	1 oz.
Flower of Sulphur	1 oz.
Glycerine	2 oz.
Sweet spirits of Nitre	1 oz.

Mix and wash.

FOR RUNNING SORES ON THE LIMBS.

Apply a poultice, for six hours, made of hop yeast and pulverized charcoal lukewarm, after that wash the sore with fresh milk. Then take pure pine tar and spread it on a piece of scorched linen, then apply it to the sore and leave it on for 9 days. When the 9 days are up then remove the cloth, greasing it first with lard or fish oil so it will remove easily. Then wash the sore with 1 pint of lukewarm soft water to which there has been added 20 drops of carbolic acid. After this dress the sore twice a day and apply cod liver oil.

FOR OLD SORES.

Ashes from good cigars and ashes from linen cloth and white chalk, equal parts of each; apply to the sore.

FRESH SORES AND ALL SORES.

| Soft Water | 1 qt. | Nut Gall powder | 1 oz. |
| Litharge | 1 oz. | White Vitriol | 2 dr. |

Wash twice a day.

FEVER IN SORES.

Bluestone in Rye Whiskey or soft water, as much as will dissolve and wash the sore.

PROUD FLESH.

Soft Water	3 oz.	Brown Sugar	1 oz.
Burnt Alum	2 dr.	Nitric Acid	2 dr.
	Sublimate	1 Sc.	

FELON.

The raw yolk of an egg and as much salt. Mix well and tie on felon from 25 to 30 minutes.

Nettle Sting resembling Erysipelas. It stings and itches. The signs are the same as Liver Complaint. Wash first with salt water, then wash with tea made from nettle and also drink some of the tea.

A Valuable Remedy for Backache and Suppressed Urine is Medicament. It may be obtained at most drug stores. Sweet Nitre is good for the urine.

RING WORM.

Place two old copper pennies, or pure copper, in two tablespoonfuls of good cider vinegar. When the vinegar is green, wash the sore twice a day.

BOILS AND CARBUNCLES.

Brown Sugar	½ lb.	Beeswax	½ lb.
Sheep Tallow	½ lb.	Honey	1 pt.

Sweet Oil, 1 gill.

SALT RHEUM.

Rock Oil	1 oz.	Opodeldoc	1 oz.
Spike Oil	1 oz.	Turpentine	1 oz.

Mix and apply twice a day. Keep a wet cold cloth on all the time.

CHAPPED HANDS AND TETTER.

Olive Oil	1 oz.	Caustic	1 dr.
Glycerine	1 oz.	Carbolic Acid	10 dr'ps.

Mix and apply twice a day.

For Poison, grease with Sweet Spirits of Nitre three times a day.

Hair in the Stomach, commonly caused by children playing with cats and dogs, thereby getting hair into the mouth. Take sugar and scraped turnip, mix and let stand for 24 hours, then use the juice. Dose: One tablespoonful three times a day. The signs are loss of appetite and health until they become very poor.

JOINT WATER.

Take a new white clay pipe and pulverize it as fine as dust and put on the sore.

For Swelling on man or beast : Take "fine cut" tobacco and make a strong tea ; wash two or three times a day.

FOR ULCERS.

| Raw Linseed Oil | 1 pt. | Sheep Tallow | ½ pt. |
| Olive Oil | ½ pt. | Beeswax | 1 lb. |

Horse Mint, 1 handful.
Mullen Flowers, 1 teacupful.
Fry and strain in the tallow and mix.

WHITE SWELLING, AND SALT RHEUM.
Etc., Etc.

Comfrey Root 2 handfuls.

Bayberry Oil	2 oz.	Sheep Tallow	4 oz.
Pine Gum	2 oz.	Beeswax	4 oz.
Rosin	2 oz.	Castile Soap	2 oz.

Fresh, Unsalted Butter 4 oz.

| Dog's Oil | 4 oz. | Sweet Oil | 4 oz. |

Pure Neat Foot Oil 4 oz.

Mix, put in a clean crock and boil one and one-half hours, continually stirring with a wooden stick and strain, then add

Tincture of Myrrh	1 oz.
Burnt Alum	1 oz.
Tincture of Camphor	1 oz.

BURNS.

Beeswax	1 pt.	Raw Linseed Oil	1 pt.
Sheep Tallow	1 pt.	Lard	1 pt.

Melt and **mix.**

ANOTHER.—Burn a piece **of** linen cloth until it is all black. Apply linseed oil on the sore, then cover with the burnt cloth. **Repeat** every two days until healed.

ANOTHER.—Sweet **Cream** ½ pt. Raw Linseed Oil ½ pt. Mix and apply to the sore.

OIL FOR BURNS.

Rye **Whiskey**	1 qt.	Camphor	1 oz.
Aloes	1 oz.	Opium	2 dr.

Mullen **flowers** 2 **handfuls,** White Lilies 1 handful.

Use externally and internally

BURNS.

Grease three times a day with cold sweet cream and keep the air from the sore, or use

Alcohol 1 pt., **Green Nettle,** stalk and leaves **1** handful. Mix: Take one tablespoonful of this and **put** it in 1 pt. of cold water. Then take white cotton batting and wet it in this water Solution. Apply to the burn and keep it wet with this Solution until all the fire is drawn out, then use Pain liniment as previously prescribed.

BURNS, SPRAINS, SWELLING, ETC.

Olive Oil	½ pt.	Soft Water	½ pt.
Alcohol	½ pt.	Borax	1 oz.
Bluestone	1 dr.	Saleratus	1 oz.

Sore from stepping in a nail. Place the foot half an hour in Rye Whiskey three times a day for three days, then use any healing salve or liniment.

SPRAINS.

Oil of Olive and as much Camphor as it will dissolve.

PAIN OR SWELLING.

Take ½ gallon strong Smart Weed tea add 1 oz. Alum and wash parts afflicted.

FEVER SWEATS.

Sweet milk 1 teacupful, add one raw egg, brandy 3 tablespoonfuls. Dose—one-half teaspoonful daily and wash daily with Saleratus water and eat all the lemons you can.

COUGH.

Tea of Red Clove Blossom is excellent.

COUGH.

Laudanum	1 tablespoonful
Wine of Ipecac	1 tablespoonful
Honey	12 tablespoonfuls
Cider Vinegar	12 tablespoonfuls

Dose: For children one teaspoonful 3 times a day.

SYRUP FOR CONSUMPTION OR COUGH.

Raw Linseed oil	½ pt.	Brandy	½ pt.
Hoarhound tea	½ pt.	Gum Arabic	1 oz.
Laudanum	½ oz.	Paregoric	2 oz.
Ipecacuan	2 dr.	Loaf Sugar	¼ lb.

Juice of boiled onions . ½ pt.

Dose: Small tablespoonful three times a day.

COUGH SYRUP.

Seven onions boiled in one quart of soft water.

Seven tablespoonfuls flax seed boiled in one pint of soft water. One handful Hoarhound boiled in one pint of soft water. Strain all and put them together, add 1 oz. of Paregoric and 1½ lb. best brown sugar and boil down to one quart. Dose: one tablespoonful three times a day.

CONSUMPTION.

Rye Whiskey	1 qt.	Squill	2 oz.
Hyssops	2 oz.	Dandelion Root	2 oz.

Put in a bottle and set in a warm place for ten days shaking it frequently. Dose: 1 tablespoonful three times a day.

COUGH MEDICINE.

Wheat bran	1 qt.	Rain Water	2 qt.

Boil and strain then add

Slippery Elm Tea	1 pt.	Lemon Oil	1 oz.

Sugar ½ lb.

Dose: One tablespoonful three times a day.

ANOTHER COUGH MEDICINE.

| Raisins | 1 lb. | Loaf Sugar | 1 lb. |
| Licorice Gum | 2 oz. | Rain Water | 2 qt. |

Mix and boil down to one quart. Dose: One tablespoonful.

DYSPEPSIA.

First keep the bowels regular and take Bi-carbonate of Soda or Potassa. Dose : One grain three times a day; or, take Carbonate of Potassa for two weeks, the size of a pea, three times a day in a little cold water, then increase the dose double after the two weeks. Eat nothing greasy and no food containing Saleratus or Baking Powder.

FLUX.

One pint warm fresh milk, taken as soon as milked, pure white glue 1 dr., and one-half tea-cupful of weeping willow leaves (if obtainable) and cook a little and drink warm, divided into three doses, morning, noon and evening, and take good ripe field corn and roast and use instead of coffee for drink.

To Stop Vomiting caused from stomach or other reasons : Take from 1 to 2 teaspoonfuls of common table salt.

RUPTURE.

Grease frequently with Bayberry oil and wear a truss until healed.

ITCH.

Take Yellow Dock root and scrape it and put in a hog bladder and bury it 24 hours in the ground. Before burying it, add to the Yellow Dock 1 lb. of lard and Flower of Sulphur 4 oz. Apply once a day.

GRAVEL.

Three tablespoonfuls of the white from chicken droppings in one pint of cider vinegar. Let stand 24 hours, shaking frequently. Strain. Dose—one tablespoonful three times a day, and then use daily a tea made from the tops of carrots and water melon seeds, sweetened with honey.

PILES.

Bitter Aloes 1 oz., in 1 pt. Rye Whiskey. Dose—one tablespoonful once a day; or,

Get Kidney Nuts and eat three a day. External, take some of the grease found on the shafts of machinery and grease the sore, or take pure fish oil,—or grease with Bayberry oil.

SICK HEADACHE.

Alcohol	½ pt.	Quinia	8 gr.
Rhubarb	10 gr.	Myrrh	10 gr.
	Capsicum	11 gr.	

Dose: 5 to 15 drops or take fine charcoal one teaspoonful in cold water.

HEADACHE AND EARACHE.

Wash the part afflicted with bay rum.

ERYSIPELAS.

Sugar of lead   1 oz. | Soft Water   ½ gal.
    Mix and wash.

SMALL POX.

Hot Rain Water 1 pt. add Cream of Tartar 1 oz.
    When cold make in three doses and take
one hour apart. Keep ordinarily cool.

SMALL POX AND SCARLET FEVER.

Sulphate of Zinc 1 gr. Foxglove (Digitalis)
1 gr. Sugar ½ teaspoonful.

Mix with two teaspoonfuls of water then
when thoroughly mixed add four ounces of
water. Take a teaspoonful every hour. Either
disease will disappear in twelve hours. For
children smaller doses according to ages.

INTERNAL AND EXTERNAL LINIMENT FOR CHOLERA, CRAMPS, ETC.

Oil of Cedar   2 dr. | Oil of Hemlock   2 dr.
Oil of Amber   2 dr. | Oil of Origanum 2 dr. .
Oil of Wormwood 3 dr. | Oil of Iodine   1 dr.
Opium   2 Sc. | Alcohol   ½ pt.

BLOOD PURIFIER.

Dandelion Root, Burdock Root, Yellow
Dock Root, of each one handful, boil in 2 qts.
soft water down to 1 qt. Dose—1 tablespoonful three times a day.

PAIN KILLER.

Myrrh 1½ oz. | Guaiacum Resin 1 oz.
Red Pepper 1 dr. | Alcohol diluted 2 pts.
Oil of Anise Seed 1 dr.

Mix and shake frequently for 5 days then filter.

PAIN KILLER.

Take one teaspoonful of Compound Powder of Jalap. Then take ½ of the powder and mix it in one gill of soft water and take internally. If necessary repeat in two or three days. This liniment is used especially for continuing pain as in Tumors, Cancers and Rheumatism.

CONTENTS.

Author's Preface.. 3
General Remarks on Cancer... 5
Seirrhus or Hard Cancer.. 7
Cancer Powder for internal use.. 9
Cancer Tea for internal use.. 9
External treatment for Cancer...11
Cancer Salve..11
Healing Salve...13
Encephaloid, Rose or Soft Cancer and treatment 15, 34
Colloid Cancer and treatment..18
Melanosis or Black Cancer and treatment...........19, 37
Epithelial or Cutaneous Cancer and treatment....20, 38
Cancer of the Stomach or Bowels......................................22
Causes of Cancers..24
Instructions to Patients..25, 35
Testimonials..27
Various Cancer Remedies..33
Good Poultices...34
To Relieve Pain...35
For Tumors...35
Salt Rheum...36, 51
For Gangrene..36
A Remedy...37
Cure for the bite of Mad Dogs and other Animals....39
A Remedy for Hydrophobia...41

VALUABLE RECEIPTS PROVED BY DR. **G. S. PETRY**
AND OTHERS.

Whooping Cough..43
Jaundice...43
Sore Eyes...43
Rheumatism or Neuralgia..43
Erysipelas, Itch, Ivy Poison, Old Sores...............................44
Felons...44, 50
Chafing in Children...44
Burns..44, 53
Run Around...44
Catarrh...44
Magic Liniment...44
Blood Purifier..45, 58
Liniments..45

Lightning Oil.... 45
Pain Liniment...46
Liniment for Sores 46
Diarrhea...47
Croup.............................. 47
Rheumatism...47
Ague.. 48
Golden Seal.................................. 48
Cholera Balm................... 48
For Cancer and other Sores......................49
All kinds of Sores....................................49
For Running Sores..49
For Fresh and Old Sores..................... 50
Fever in Sores..50
Proud Flesh...50
Nettle Sting......................... 50
A Valuable Remedy......................................50
Ring Worm...51
Boils and Carbuncles.................................51
Chapped hands and Tetter.................. 51
For Poison..51
Hair in the Stomach 51
Joint Water..52
For Swelling... 52
For Ulcers...52
White Swelling, Salt Rheum, etc.,........................52
Burns, Sprains, Swelling, etc.,...............................54
Fever Sweats................................ 54
Cough... 54
Syrup for Consumption or Cough.................. 55
Cough Medicine...55
Another Cough Medicine......................................56
Dyspepsia.. ...56
Flux...56
To Stop Vomiting.............. 56
Rupture... 56
Itch 57
Gravel..57
Piles..57
Sick Headache...57
Erysipelas..58
Small Pox and Scarlet Fever...............................58
Liniments for Cholera, Cramps, etc.,.......................58
Pain Killer...59